LIBERATE YOUR BEHIND

Trace Williams

Cover design by Joleene Naylor

Editing by Trace Williams

Editor Disclaimer

This Ebook is dedicated to the memory of

Lily

who died much too young,

best friend to my daughter Shannon

TABLE OF CONTENTS

PREFACE

This is a Revolutionary book! First of a kind! At the same time it is also a Satire as it exposes our foolishness and sheepish Capitalist behavior. It's also an Environmental book for the wanton destruction of our precious environment (virgin trees cut and toxic chemicals used to process the raw pulp) and electrical energy waste, not to mention the excess waste product that our sewage processing plants must contend with. It is also an Educational book in that it teaches you about learned behavior and to be a better steward of the environment, think for yourself, be creative and recycle. And finally, it is a Financial book in that it teaches you to save up to 400 dollars a year per family to better use towards your kids, yourself, even your retirement!

It took a serious illness (Cancer) 6 years ago for me to discover and learn what is covered in this book. Through the following years, I have evolved this simple System through trial and error and further experimentation. However, when I had the Cancer, I was slowly going broke financially and basically surviving on a bread maker, cheap margarine, and little else. I lost just about everything and was struggling to make rent and save money anywhere I could find. One day, I found myself in the grocery store and buying my margarine when I remembered I was low on toilet paper. I got angry and thought how stupid it is that I have to pay money each time I go to the bathroom to wipe my behind! Also, how expensive this paper on a roll had become, especially since I could not afford even my food. Yes, you read it correctly, the Smelly topic no one talks about except the multi-nationals making 100's of millions every time we need to relieve ourselves. You see them with their cute Ads all claiming to be the softest, longest lasting, and guarantying the cleanest result! Some even include childish Bears and Kittens all in the great attempt to make you laugh, gain greater confidence, and market share, while continuing to damage our planet and yes.....keep you stupid and in the dark! By the way, they never thank you for the Billions of unnecessary dollars they take from you nor will they educate you on environmentally friendly alternatives!

So get ready to enter inside the forbidden/taboo world of **Toilet Paper.** You are about to learn the history of wiping your behind, the flush toilet, the history, enormous industry size and damage caused by Big toilet paper companies, the clean future ahead, and my revolutionary replacement system, which in the meantime, saves you money each month, is so easy to implement and saves our precious environment today and into the future. Welcome to my **Towelette System** of keeping cleaner. Come along my journey of discovery, personal challenge and growth. It's finally time to liberate your behind!

Back to top

CHAPTER 1

History of toilet paper and what people used before its introduction

The history of wiping our behinds has come a long way since ancient times. The Greeks were said to use stones and even pieces of clay! I sure hope for them, those stones were rounded…ouch! Yes, today, our toilet paper gets taken for granted as the "go-to" system for clean behinds. In pr-historic times, it is likely cave men and women used both stones and leaves for their daily function. The ancient Chinese were fond of using straw and also pieces of broken pottery. Again. Ouch!

The Romans took their daily function a lot more leisurely! They had public facilities in each town where everyone went to do their duty. Public latrines date back to the 2nd century B.C. Long marble benches were set up in Public Bath houses with holes cut into them at a certain distance from each other. There were no dividers or individual benches; you could find yourself sitting next to your neighbor or even the lady down the street. Romans used a sea sponge on the end of a short stick. The sponge stick was then returned to a central basin filled with sea water, water and even vinegar at times. Sometimes, in front of you were smaller holes set up to rest your long stick . So your sponge on a stick was your toilet paper. After use, it went back into the central basin where it laid in a sea water . Everyone shared like good Romans and there was little concern for germs as the salt water was your disinfectant. The Romans believed in sharing and everyone else was welcome to your sponge stick once you were finished. Once you were through, it was customary to fill a clay jar with water and pour it by way of the front of your bench to help flush the stools on their merry way to the river via pipes made of lead and clay. So not only did you have to scrub yourself clean with a sea salt sponge, you also were obligated to getting your stools on their way.

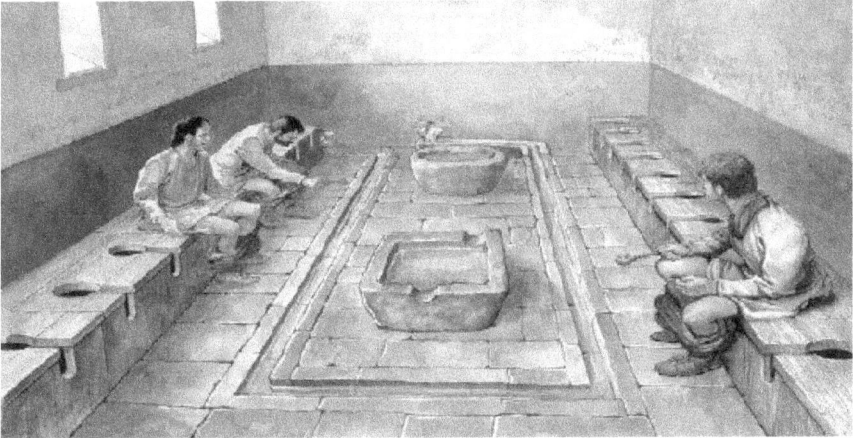

Note that the Romans never dried their behinds! They simply scrubbed their behinds and likely rinsed their sponge for one last wipe. Once they completed this step, they lowered their toga and air dried their wetness away.

The Chinese used a dry system of straw, leaves and broken pieces of pottery which must have hurt badly! The reason was simple; the Chinese recycled their stools as fertilizer which while efficient often led to dysentery and other disease. There was also an industry based around collecting people's stools and selling them to large scale farmers as fertilizer. Talk about a smelly business...literally!

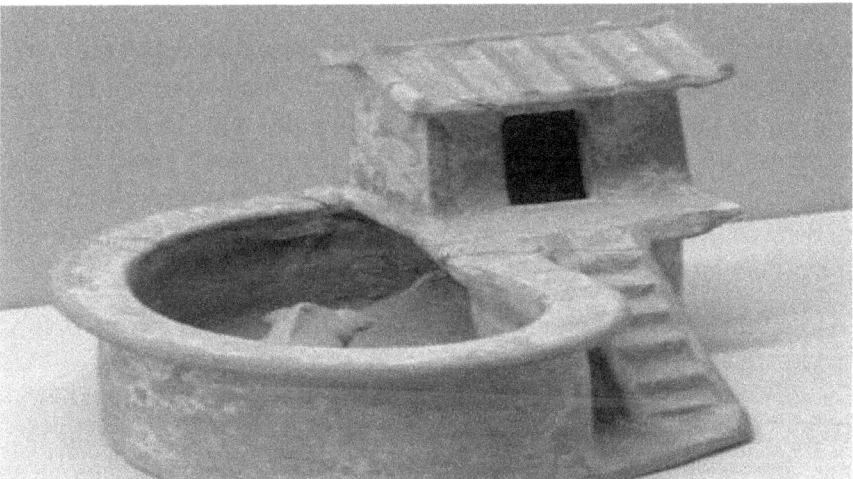

In the above Han Dynasty (100 A.D) illustration of an outhouse, we can see that the person simply climbed to the edge, then slightly squatted and let it drop into the pit below. In the pit were pigs which ate the stools and got fat for much later human consumption. Under the Tang Dynasty (7th century) , business people in China started to build pay toilets. These toilets were mud brick made for one person the size of a bathroom stall today, with a hole in the floor to squat over. Businesses collected the poop from these pay toilets and used donkey carts to pull cartloads of poop out to the country. Farmers bought the poop to spread on their fields. Most city people didn't want to pay for toilets and so used clay pots in their own houses for later dumping in street or river close to them. Sometime around 500 A.D, rich people in China started to use the very first paper to wipe themselves. Most people could not afford fancy toilet paper and went on using whatever was at hand. Slowly, random paper products soon became more popular for their comfort and softness. Around 1391, the great Emperor Hongwu (Ming Dynasty) decreed that large 2 X 3 foot paper sheets must be made for his toilet time.

The Vikings were said to have used Wool to wipe themselves. The Eskimo/Inuit used snow in Winter and moss during the Summers. In the Southern reaches, many used coconut husk which is fibrous.

In the era of Colonial America, things were not much more advanced. Patriots and their families were often found using whatever was at hand which included even dried corn cobs! It was not until much later that they realized they could use discarded print material, papers and newspapers of the day. It was not until the catalogue era that Americans started using old Catalogue pages. Catalogue manufacturers conveniently cut holes through the top corner of the catalogues and farmers almanacs so they could be hung on a string in the outhouse. They knew people had time on the toilet to browse their goods. Now you will look at your bathroom reading material a little differently knowing this.

While this is a book on toilet paper, the industry around it and my newer cleaner, more environmentally responsible "Towelette System" of personal hygiene, I want to give honorary mention to the both the inventors of the modern toilet and the flushing mechanism that goes with it. While many believe the Brit Thomas Crapper was the inventor of both, this is incorrect. Although a successful Plumber during the mid 1800's, Crapper's accomplishment also include 9 patents for plumbing innovations during his lifetime, 3 of them consisting of improvements to the flushing part of a toilet's operation. He is also credited with opening one of the first bathroom showrooms in 1870. Credit for the invention of the toilet in 1596 goes to Brit Sir John Harington (16th century Courtier) who not only conceived the toilet idea but also built and installed an early prototype in the palace of Queen Elizabeth I, his Godmother.

That's why it commonly called "the John" and not so much the Crapper! Before this in England, you used what you had on hand, likely old rags and newspaper and collected your waste in a chamber pot for convenient dumping in the street or the Thames river nearby if you lived in London. It is said to have gotten so bad in the mid 1800's that Parliament had to recess in the Summer due to the Great Stink coming out of the Thames. Now if you were the King or Queen, you had a special servant called the "Groom of the Stool." A highly respected position, this servant of the Crown would take care of the head of State with hands on attention.

Toilet paper as we know it was first invented in Massachusetts USA by Joseph Gayetty in 1857 and marketed in December of that same year. His new toilet paper was composed of flat sheets of pure Manila Hemp and contained Aloe as a lubricant and much better than the old catalogue pages Brits and Americans were used to. 1000 sheets cost you 1 dollar which was big money back then. Gayetty even had his new toilet paper watermarked with his name and New York on it. Marketed as "Gayetty's Medicated Paper For The Water-Closet" (bathroom of today), he was attacked as a Quack by the New Orleans Medical News and Hospital Gazette in 1859. This stemmed from the fact he claimed it as an anti-hemorrhoid medical product. Gayetty claimed his invention was also the "Greatest Necessity of the Age" and warned against the perils of using toxic inked old catalogue pages to wipe your behind. More than a hundred years later, Gayetty was so right. Not only did he invent modern toilet paper, he was the first to join forces with a large paper company (Diamond Mills Paper) to produce and help market his product way into the future which continues today and is a multi-billion dollar industry! He further joined forces with big business in 1866 when he entered into a 10 year marketing contract with Demas Barnes and Company to vend and sell in his name.

The first patent issued for perforated toilet paper sheets went to New York business man Seth Wheeler. Wheeler, who was also the owner of the Albany Perforated Wrapping Sheet Company, is said to have invented the way toilet paper is created and used in this way.

In 1867, Edward, Thomas and Clarence Scott, all brothers from Philadelphia were the first to successfully **market** perforated toilet paper on a larger scale. They sold their new rolls from a push cart and this was the beginning of the giant Scott Paper Company! Apparently, they were so ashamed of the business they were in that they never put their name on their paper rolls or liked to talk shop with family and friends.

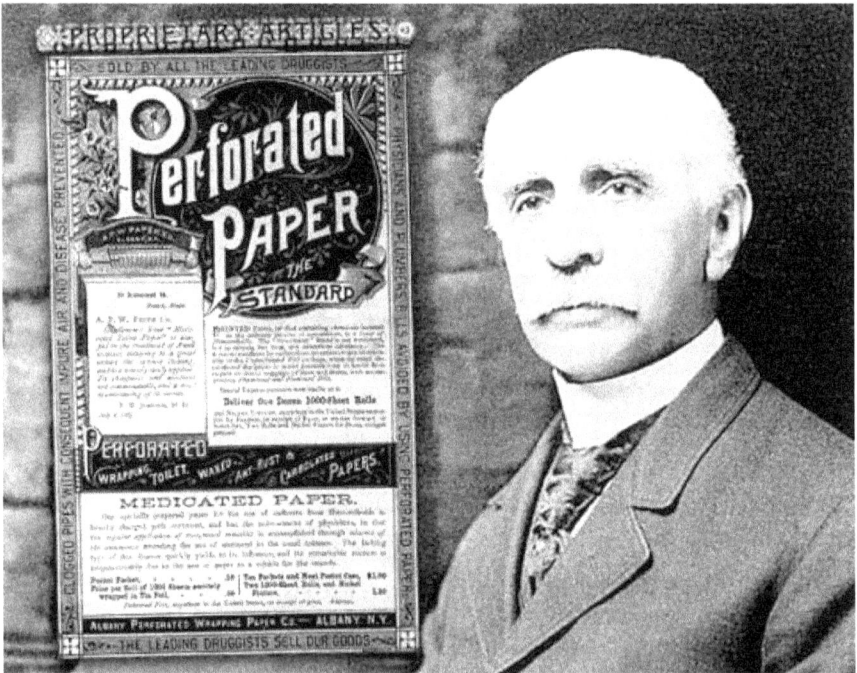

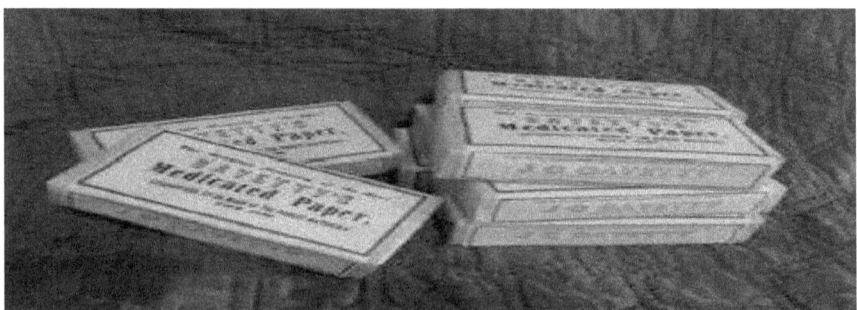

Above pictures showing Mr. Gayetty with an advertisement from the time period and how Gayetty toilet paper was purchased. As can be seen, the paper came in separate sheets of 1000.

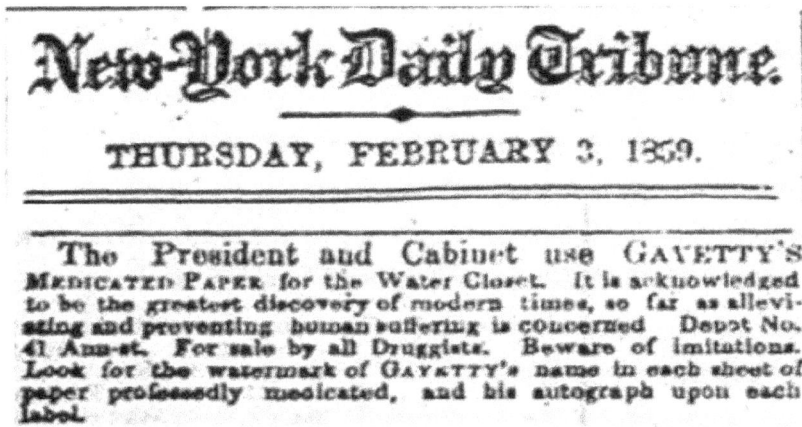

New-York Daily Tribune.

THURSDAY, FEBRUARY 3, 1859.

The President and Cabinet use GAYETTY'S MEDICATED PAPER for the Water Closet. It is acknowledged to be the greatest discovery of modern times, so far as allevi-ating and preventing human suffering is concerned Depot No. 41 Ann-st. For sale by all Druggists. Beware of imitations. Look for the watermark of GAYETTY's name in each sheet of paper professedly medicated, and his autograph upon each label.

As can be seen in the above picture, Gayetty claimed that the very President of United States and Cabinet used his new toilet paper invention.

By 1935, it was all about Big Business and marketing strategy. Quilted Northern (formerly Northern Tissue), advertised that their toilet paper was "Splinter Free." Still in the multi-billion dollar multi-ply industry today, it's obvious their claim was a success as demand sky-rocketed over the decades. Today, Americans alone are said to use over 7 billion rolls of toilet paper each year!

The current era is all about marketing Superior claims and increasing market share from competitors in a mature market! Softest, strongest, most economical price, more sheets per roll, family size packs, and of course most superior clean with ripples and grooves. It is also said that firms are squeezing profits from creating smaller sheets. It's Super Big Business (a giant industry) and let's now take a closer look in Chapter 2.

Back to top

Toilet paper economics…Big Business & Bigger Damage to Our Environment

On average, Americans use 57 sheets of toilet paper a day, amounting to 27 rolls per year! The estimate is Americans alone use over **7 Billion** rolls of toilet paper per year! That's **27,000** trees a day that go down the toilet as waste paper! This is horrible considering that some 40% of all toilet rolls sold in the UK and 98% in America are made from paper derived from virgin forests. Sadly, while toilet paper can be made at similar cost from recycled paper fibre, it is the fibre from live trees that help give it a plush feel. In an eye-opening video, InsuranceQuotes.org takes a look at the true economic, environmental and health costs of the $30 billion toilet paper industry worldwide. Americans alone spend a total of **$6-7 billion** per year on toilet paper, depending on the source.

Average annual expenditure on cleansing and toilet tissue, paper towels and napkins per consumer unit in the United States from 2007 to 2015 (in U.S. dollars)*

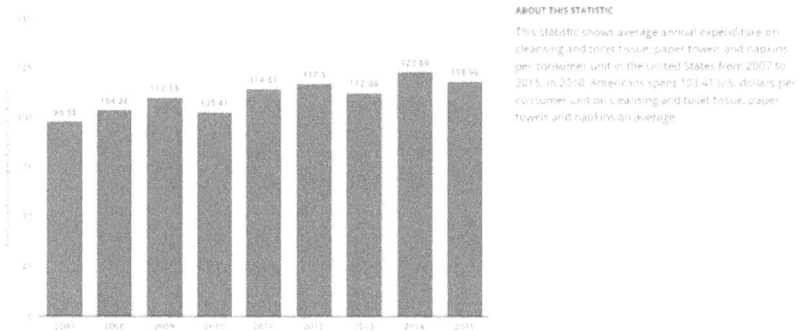

As can be seen, Americans are spending over 100 dollars per individual on paper products including toilet paper. About half of this is directly for toilet paper. I believe this is an underestimate as I can easily use 7-12 dollars per month depending on the Brand and quality I buy. It is currently believed that 25-30% of the world's population currently uses toilet paper.

Not only is toilet paper environmentally damaging to produce, recycled toilet paper has been found to contain small amounts of

Bisphenol A (BPA), which is known to be linked to Cancer, infertility and heart disease. Research shows that **Bidets or Towelette's** are cleaner and less likely to result in vaginitis, urinary tract infections and more. If those 27,000 trees cut down a year were left standing, they could have absorbed 9.9 million miles of car driving CO2 created. Sadly, toilet paper demand is rising in China and Europe. In Canada, revenue from the toilet paper market amounted to 1.24 Billion in 2018. Canadians use on average 100 rolls per year! The market is expected to grow annually by 3.7%. China is the leader in toilet paper consumption. In 2018, the revenue generated from toilet paper sales in China was a whopping 15.3 Billion US dollars! In the US today, the toilet paper industry is dominated by 3 manufacturers: Georgia Pacific, Procter & Gamble and Kimberly Clark, with the latter generating 2.14 billion US dollars in 2016. Private label brands accounted for 1.7 billion in 2017 alone. These were likely manufactured by the big 3. As of 2017, Charmin Ultra Soft was the leading brand with just over 1 billion in US sales alone. In Canada, Kruger Products has 36.8% of the market share while Irving controls just over 21% (2016).

The real growth in the industry is happening in developing countries. There, it's booming. Toilet paper revenues in Brazil alone have more than doubled since 2004. The radical upswing in sales is believed to be driven by a combination of changing demographics, social expectations, and rising disposable income.

The truth here is that Toilet paper, even dressed up toilet paper with cute kittens and bears on the packaging is an Environmental Nightmare and Crime! Forget the measly plastic straw…nothing is killed to make plastic! It's bad too but toilet paper is really bad news. In today's age of carbon footprint awareness, the mere idea of killing millions of trees yearly should be offensive. It takes an estimated 39 gallons of water to make 1 roll of toilet paper! It's an antiquated solution to our daily function. And **Eco** labels are NO guarantee the forests are being protected as the Canadian Broadcasting Corporation (CBC) reported in 2012. The problem lies in the fact that large paper companies are still clear cutting areas and only replanting with one species like Spruce. As a result, forest diversity is lost and what grows up is virtually a tree farm not a true forest. Critics claim that government forest policy along with poor management and corporate greed are the driving forces which are to blame.

In 2009, Greenpeace issued its first national guide for American consumers that rates toilet tissue brands on their environmental soundness. They wanted consumers to start switching to toilet paper with recycled fibres. The fact is, no forest of any type should be cut down to make toilet paper! Currently, tissue from 100% recycled fibres makes us less than 2% of sales for at-home brands. In Europe and Latin America, products with recycled content make up 20% of the market on average. We need to nurture similar interest in North America for those who feel they cannot convert to a better system (eg.Towelette or clip on bidet) Not only is less water used to produce toilet paper from recycled fibres but also produces less paper waste that would normally go to our landfills and conserves our forests. Currently, environmental groups say 50% of the pulp used to make toilet paper in North America comes from older second growth forests that serve as important absorbents of carbon dioxide. And even worse, some is said to come from the last virgin forests which are an irreplaceable habitat.

Back to top

CHAPTER 3

Inspiration from the Indian Model

"Additionally, we don't use those chair like toilet seats. We use the one that looks like a hole in the floor. It forces you to *squat and exercise your prostate. Results in fast defecation, less chances of prostate cancer, less risk of communicable diseases, lesser hemorrhoids and stronger knees(Quora, Vicas Vimal,2016)*"

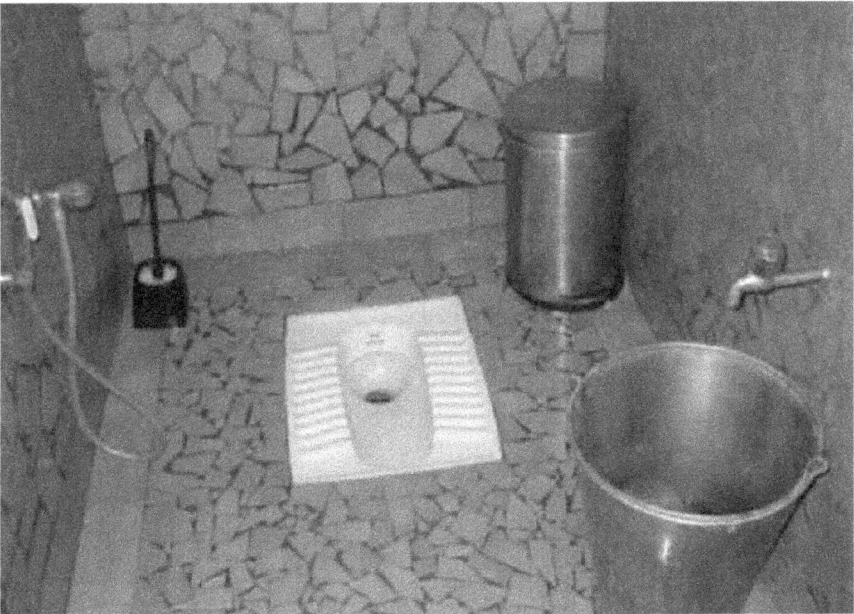

Here you have it, my inspiration for my **Towelette System**. Your probably shocked as most North Americans cannot even imagine such a toilet exists! Squat toilets are used all over the world, but are particularly common in many Asian and African countries and those with a large proportion of people of Muslim or Hindu faith who also practise anal cleansing with water. When I had Cancer and could not even afford toilet paper, I saw my first picture of this type of toilet and read a story about how trees were precious in India and they truly believed it more hygiene to clean themselves with water after soaping their behind. While some of the more modern ones are flush tank operational, most traditional ones simply have a tap nearby for rinsing after use. These peoples simply squat, have their bowel movement, soap their orifice and then rinse. Yes, some simply rinse well and don't even dry off, just like the Romans practised. For Seniors and the Disabled, a small chair with shortened legs can be placed over the squat toilet and a hole cut out in the centre. In the old days, they used ashes to clean their hands and then rinsed them. It's obvious our toilets were not designed for squatting. Also, our water taps are not very close by. However, it did get me thinking that toilet paper is wholly unnecessary as our Indian friends have proved for centuries. I then gathered all my creative juices and started my journey to totally liberate my behind without having to get rid of my North American toilet. No one should have to spend money to clean themselves after each bowel movement for something that is not optional and comes naturally! Additionally, I was disturbed by all the damage to our environment caused by toilet paper production.

Back to top

CHAPTER 4

My Towelette System

This chapter revolves around my creation of the revolutionary Towelette System for cleaning oneself after defecation. But first, I want to talk a bit about the Psychology of toilet paper use. In my introduction I talked about how we are like sheep as we do not question our love with toilet paper. Are we totally to blame? No-sadly, learned behavior is often highly trusted and stubbornly ingrained. From the time we are 2 years of age, we are toilet training with our loving parents and inherit this antiquated solution which they also inherited and so it is ingrained within us from a very young age. We don't question this and trust in our parents love for us. It certainly does not help that the industry markets this horrible product with lovable bears and kittens and appeals to your soft side with respect to comfort as well. Not to mention the toilet roll holder (courtesy of New Yorker Seth Wheeler who in 1891 had it patented) prominently in our face and always screaming replace me! Nevertheless, more people need to see the very dark side of this product. Currently in the Provinces of New Brunswick and Nova Scotia, Canada, there are huge forest clear cuts that will only be planted as future tree farms. Huge amounts of resources: water, electricity, and poisonous chlorine are used to make it white and appealing. In an age of questioning our own carbon foot we must start thinking **more for ourselves** Populations are too large now to continue rationalizing such an environmentally damaging paper product on a massive scale! I admit, it was only because of my Cancer and poverty that I came to this position in life. I realize that many of us have busy lives and need a little help. That's why I wrote this ebook, to inspire you and give you all my knowledge of 5 years experimentation and evolution. I know what works best and below I am going to show you how to free yourself from Big Paper! It's cheap to do and anyone can afford some soap, an old towel and a rubber glove! I wrote the other chapters to give you insight into how we got here, the monster generational society helped create and operates behind curtains today, and the promising clean future ahead

I want you also to save money yearly and feel good about saving mother earth and our precious resources of electricity, water, and trees. The most important paragraph in this whole book is this:

<u>"Only we can Stop this run-away toilet paper roll! We must as a society understand it's an Environmental crime and immediately STOP using it! Only then will we choke out production if no one further buys it."</u>

My system is beautiful in its simplicity and the freedom it gives me and those who are willing to give it a go. It's been 5 years since I implemented the system in my own bathroom. Some aspects of the system have changed and evolved over time but the fundamental parts remain the same. Hence, the name Towelette, since as you have likely guessed, small Towelette's make up the heart of the system. Unlike messy toilet paper which is a dry system, my system is a wet system which requires water like the Indian squatting toilet. In the early days, I tried to use the towelette's dry just like toilet paper and then folded them for laundering. Since I did not want to just throw them in dirty with my other laundry items, I experimented with filling tin containers like the ones sold with fancy Scotch bottles full of a concoction of vinegar, Mr.Clean, Pine Sol, Bleach and of course water. This made one heck of a strong disinfecting solution and I simply placed the folded towelette's in there and dumped the whole container in the washer for cleaning. At that time we still had one of those mechanical washers so it was no big deal. I certainly didn't need to add any laundry soap as it was a strong enough combination of cleaners. However, they had to be cleaned weekly and it was a pain remembering to clean my towelette's in that tin container. Also, I had to bring the whole container from upstairs to the basement and there was always the hazard of falling and making a mess(even with a lid on). Over time I realized this won't continue to work as not only was it inconvenient for cleaning, I was worried about families with young kids and knew this would not work as a family friendly system. During this time I also experimented with different pattern styles and sizes for my towelette's. While some people use old flannel for their construction, I choose old bath towel material for its strength, softness and long lasting use. I cut this towel into the following shapes: 14 inch toilet paper like lengths, a triangular napkin type design, small squares, 9 inch toilet like lengths, small square design and 11X7 inch rectangular design style. Immediately it was apparent that what works for paper toilet paper does not work for cloth towelette style wipes. The human hand naturally felt most comfortable using the 11"X7" rectangular towelette's during the act of wiping. Additionally, the rectangular towelette could be folding after wiping and subsequently used to wipe the toilet area. You will notice that many of my towelette's are badly frayed. If you are good with a sewing machine, you can hem your towelette's so this wont happen over time. This mostly happens in the Dryer and fibres will end up on other clothes items if you choose not to hem them. I personally don't care as it's a minor consequence for all the benefits I get.

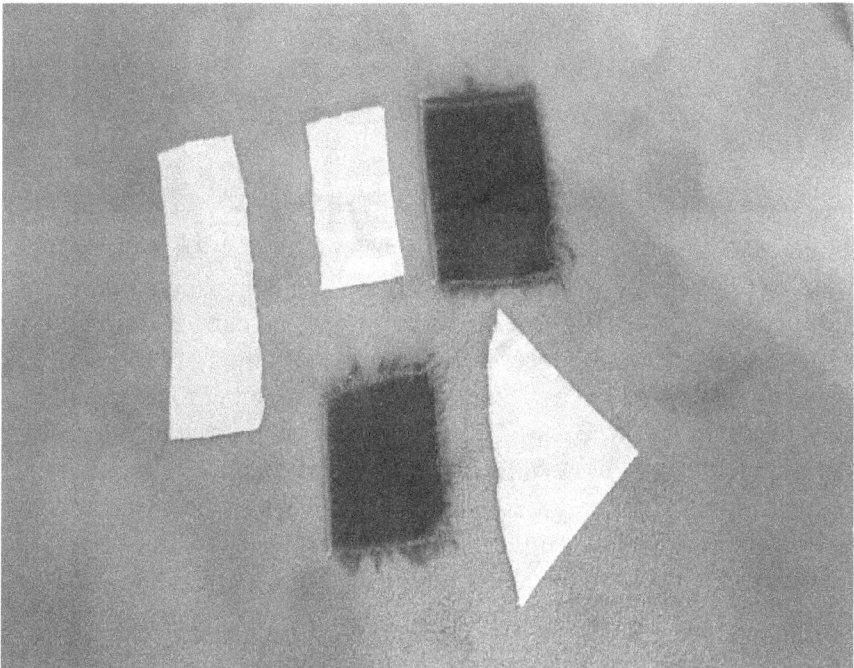

The white towelette's are a recreation for this ebook as I ceased using them awhile back. Try to use a good quality 100% cotton towel to make your 11X7 inch towelette's for best long term results.

Now we are in the heart of things. Please take a close look at the picture below. In it, you will see everything you need to make your own Towelette System a success.

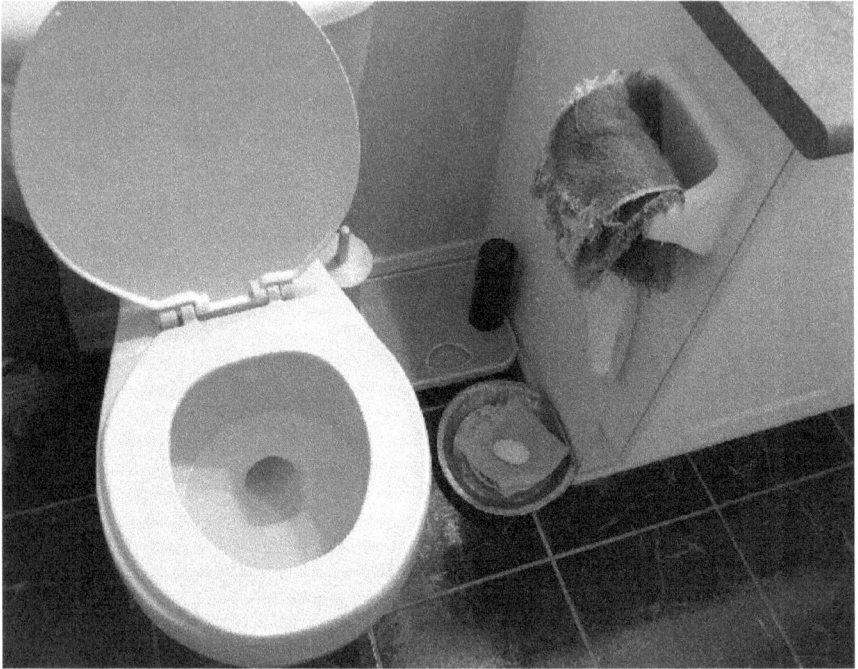

In the above picture of my actual washroom, you will see the Dove soap bar. It lies in a simple tea cup holder. To help absorb water from each use, I also have it on a small rag. You can also use a pie plate as above to catch excess drip from your hanging rubber glove. You can be as creative as you choose, just remember to keep your area clean. In my Process #2, I have eliminated soap, its holder and the pie plate pan simplifying and adding additional benefits in the process. In its place is liquid dispenser soap. So the fundamentals in your system can be as simple as a set of 10 towelette's per person/week, rubber glove, and liquid soap dispenser. That;s it!

I advise you to cut at least 10 towelette's for each adult adhering to your new system. As I don't have young children anymore, you could make smaller ones for them and start with the same number. You can use Wheeler's toilet roll holder to hold your own towelette's. This way, you won't see it empty and feel the need to replace it constantly with paper Keep your leftover rolls stored away in the linen closet and use only for guests sleeping over. Next you will need a reliable soap. Considering where it's being used, it can get pretty nasty if you choose the wrong soft brands. Discoloration and early disintegration are soaps worst enemies when used for your system. I have found that Dove works the best…not only is it the perfect size for sticking in your private area, it also appears to get harder as it ages. It will crack a bit on the edges as it slowly wears and show some nasty darker lines but overall it's your best choice to start. Let's now look at the process of which I will explain two similar routines.

In the first process, you sit on your toilet and do your natural thing. Once you feel you are finished, you simply flush without doing anything else. Now because we are not in India where water is close by and you don't have to get off your toilet, you simply use the fresh water now in your toilet from after flushing to get clean. Now get on your rubber dish washing glove (left hand only preferred), grab your bar of soap and dip it in the fresh toilet water and scrub yourself for 5-10 seconds. When you are finished, dip the soap back into the toilet water, rinse it and replace in your holder. Try not to lose your soap bar as its not fun fishing for it when your on the toilet unclean! This does happen and this along with drip is why I prefer process number 2 which follows. Now place your rubber hand back in the toilet water and gently begin rinsing your soapy bottom. You will know when the soap is gone by feel and once this happens, simply remove your rubber glove and hang it back on your nail or hook. Now grab one of your towelette's and wipe your bottom dry. Be sure to wipe with towelette fully open. There is no mess now as the soap and rinse has done the hard work. Now fold your towelette in half and wipe underneath the toilet seat and top of toilet rim. That's it, you have beaten Big Paper and saving money and the world! You can then throw your folded towelette in a bag or laundry container and wash with your cloths. If your worried about germs, buy some Lysol laundry detergent and add to your wash. I have never had any problem as you are not smearing your behind clean as with toilet paper. There is no residue, the towelette simply does the drying! I do however advise you to buy a bottle of Lysol spray and spray the top and underneath of your toilet seat as well as the top rim. This is because of drip and light spray during the scrubbing and removal of soap bar to it holder. Process number 2 eliminates the drip issue and having to look at your discolored soap cracks as it ages.

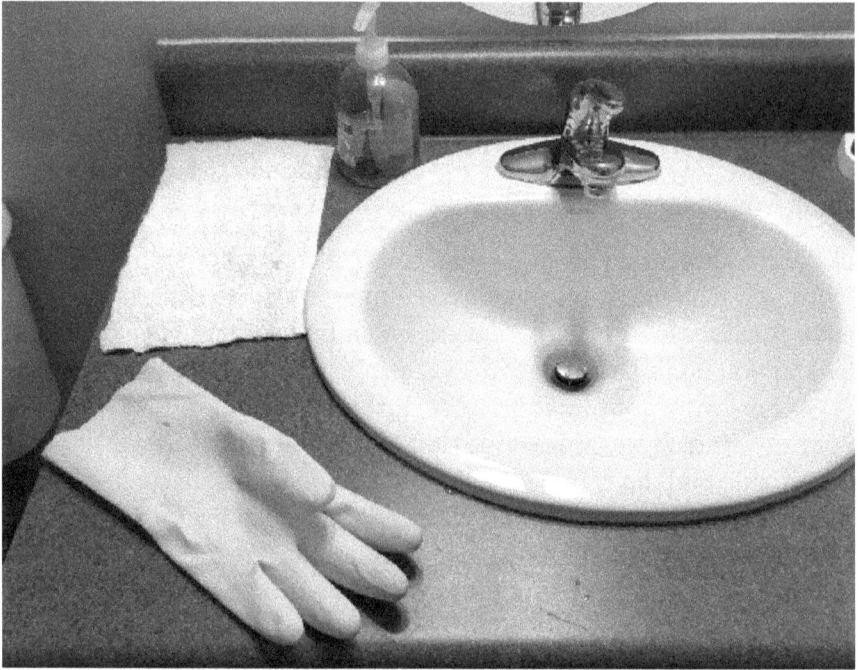

That's it… your total system, the essentials you need to need to liberate your behind! A $2 US investment that will greatly benefit the world! I also advise you buy a Lysol spray bottle for maximum disinfection of your toilet after each bowel movement.

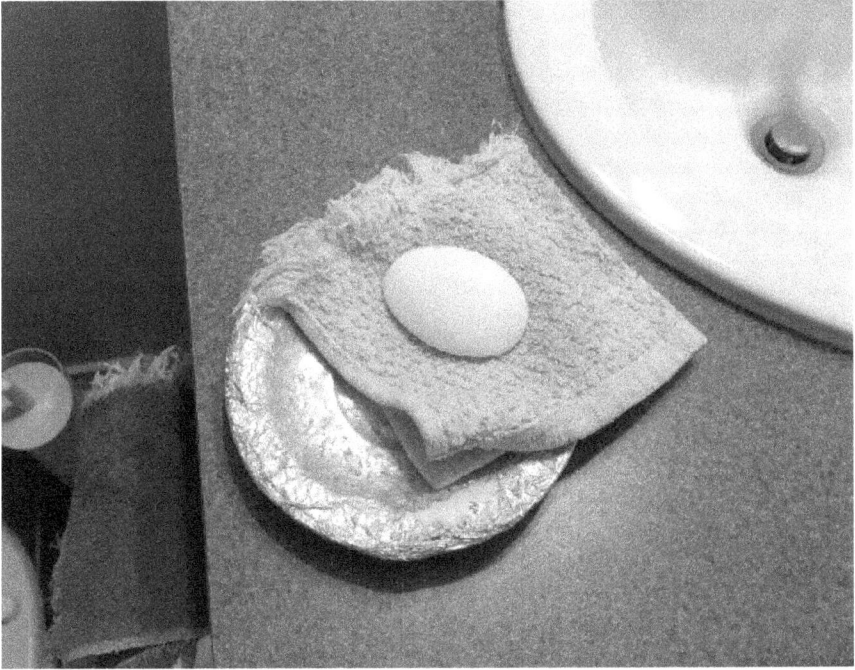

By choosing Dove, you can go months on one bar as it wears slowly and actually keeps hard! I have switch now to liquid soap as it eliminates much of the toilet spray and almost all of the drip problem created when returning the bar to its holder. The cream in Dove is also good for your sensitive skin in that area.

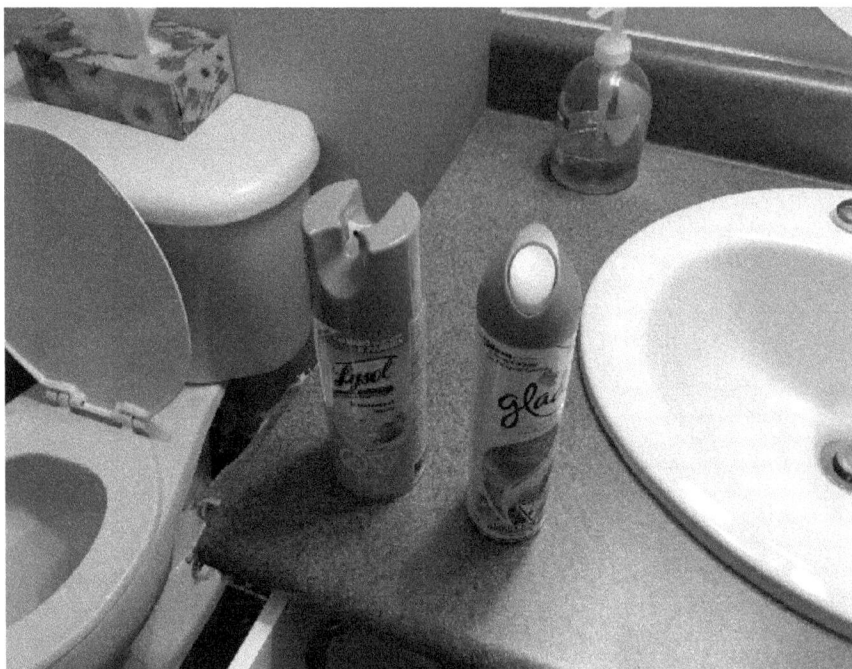

Once I wipe the top of the toilet seat and underneath, I then also wipe off the top rim of the toilet itself. Then I take my Lysol and spray all those areas. You should also wipe the soap path to its holder and spray the floor. You want to keep your towelette system very clean.

Process number 2 is simply a cleaner modified version of process number 1. Once again, you do your thing and then flush when you truly finished. Now put on your glove and take your liquid soap dispenser and give it one press. Take this liquid soap on your glove and scrub your private area for 5-10 seconds. Once complete, rinse your glove in the fresh water below and begin rinsing your bottom. Don't worry about the fecal residue…it becomes trapped in the soap and your bottom will be squeaky clean in 5-10 seconds of rinsing. If you worried about it, flush your residue and continue using water from the new flush to finish rinsing. It helps if you have a water saving toilet but considering it takes 39 gallons of water to make one stupid roll of toilet paper, I think it's a wonderful trade off in favour of our environment. Now let your rubber glove drip off for 2-3 seconds and replace on holder or nail. You can now use a dedicated larger towel for drying or your towelette. If using a towelette, wipe down your toilet sitting area top and underneath and also the top porcelain rim and place in laundry or separate basket. If your using a larger dedicated towel for drying your area, you only use your towelette for wiping clean your toilet areas and floor. You large towel can be used for up to a week before needing cleaning. Individual towelette's are to be used only once! It's now time to spray down your toilet cover, underneath it and the toilet porcelain rim with Lysol. You can also spray your glove or wash it weekly if you overly concerned. This method has no chance of losing your soap in the toilet and much less scrub spray and drip from having to replace the hard soap in its holder

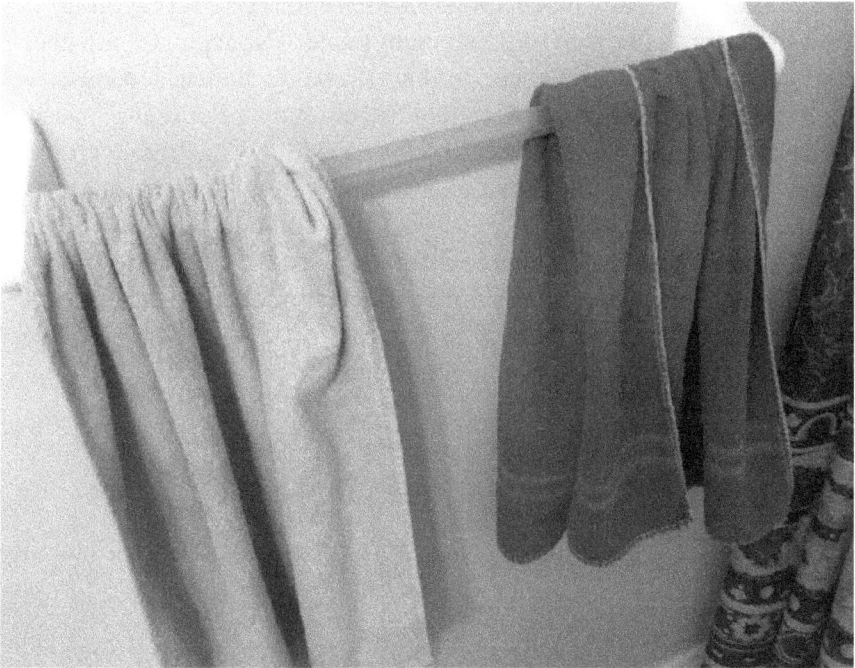

My dedicated large towel to the right and my bath towel left. Remember, your liquid soap and light scrubbing with glove on does the cleaning! Virtually no residue exists after you rinse! Your towel simply gently dries you. Nevertheless, wash it weekly with your regular laundry for total cleanliness.

Back to top

CHAPTER 5

The Clean Future: paperless toilets & clip-on Bidets

In this final chapter we are going to look at the final high tech solutions(at much greater cost of course) with regards to our age old problem of wiping our behind. As most of you know, Japan is a very ancient country with a population of 127 million (2016) and a very small land area of only 377,982 km squared. As such, resources are at a premium and advanced solutions are required for everything from household garbage to personal hygiene. The Japanese are also very industrious and advanced in their thinking. Hence, Japanese toilet bowl engineers have designed the ultimate toilet that bypasses the need for toilet paper. It's called the **Washlet.** This high tech paperless toilet delivers both a clean and dry posterior thanks to its cleaning wand and heated blow dryer. Newer models have a built-in deodorizer, which uses a charcoal filter to circulate the air in the toilet bowl. This new toilet is not so much about delivering convenience but rather their answer to the fact that using toilet paper has been declared an environmental crime!

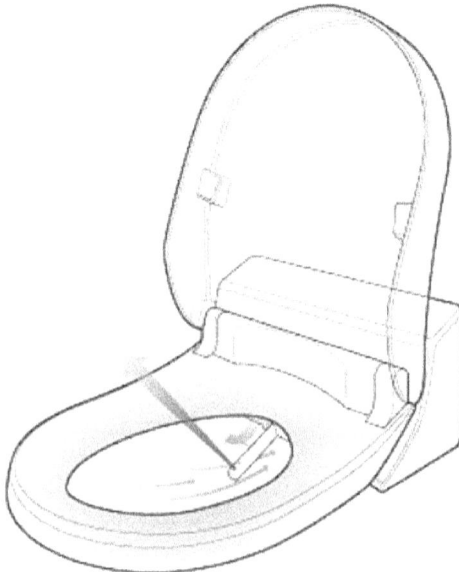

The Washlet shoots bubbled water at the user's bottom to achieve a new level of hygiene, Japanese manufacture Toto claims. This high tech toilet comes with retracting self-cleaning wand, warm air dryer and heated seat.

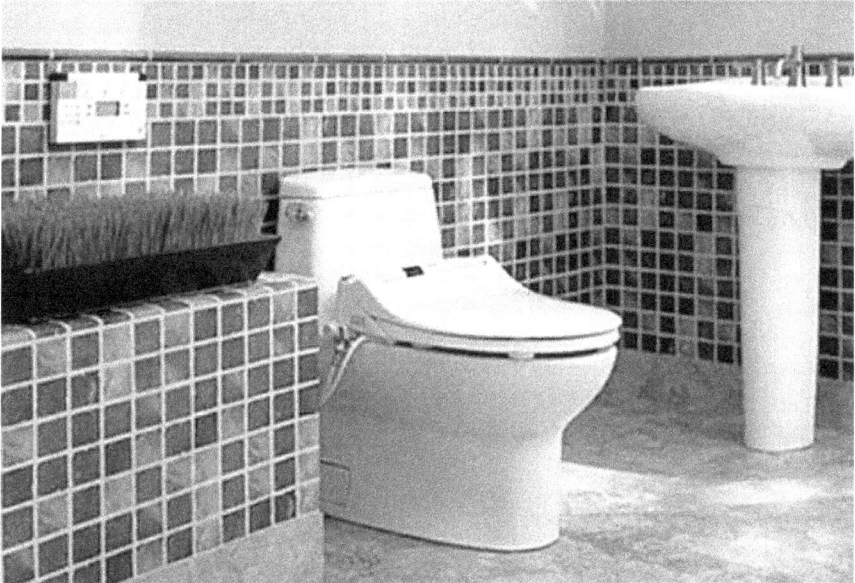

Toto claims that the Washlet is designed to introduce you to a level of unprecedented comfort, while delivering maximum cleanliness. At your command, an integrated, self-cleaning nozzle extends to release a warm and soothing stream of bubbly water, providing the maximum in personal hygiene. Once you are clean, the Washlet's wand retracts into its housing where it cleans itself, making it ready and fresh for the next user. Then the user can trip the blower which has 3 temperature settings on the high end model. In Japan, some 70% of households already own one of these. Due to its unique flush, the Washlet also uses only half (6 litres) the water compared to a traditional toilet. It also boasts a special non-stick glaze which means no harsh chemicals are needed to clean it. Apparently, a Dutch made version of this toilet is now available in the UK and I have read rave reviews. A Japanese restaurant (Saki) in London was the first UK business to install a rival version of this toilet in 2006. It is said, where installed, that people look forward to going back and using it again. No wonder the Japanese view the use of toilet paper as odd, out-dated and wasteful. Currently, price is the major deterrent for purchase and use in North America. This toilet above currently costs $2,641 US dollars and likely you will need to have one shipped over from the UK or Japan. Compare that with about 200US dollars for an average toilet in North America.

Let us now look at a low cost alternative to the above high-tech and expensive Japanese Washlet.

The **Clip-on Bidet** could spell the end of 'barbaric' wiping with antiquated toilet paper! In a bid to change our bathroom habits, Miki Agrawal originally from Montreal, Canada, has invented a mini Bidet-like device which clips onto most toilets. The compact product, named **Tushy**, is designed to clean your orifice by shooting a jet of water where needed. Agrawal claims the Tushy can be installed in only 10 minutes without the need for a professional plumber or electrician. Users first need to remove their toilet seat, fit the device to the left-hand side - which has a pipe for the jet of water positioned at the back of the seat - and finally connect it to the water supply.

'It sprays a precise jet of water exactly where you need it, and leaves you feeling clean and refreshed,' Agrawal told journalist Emma Johnson.

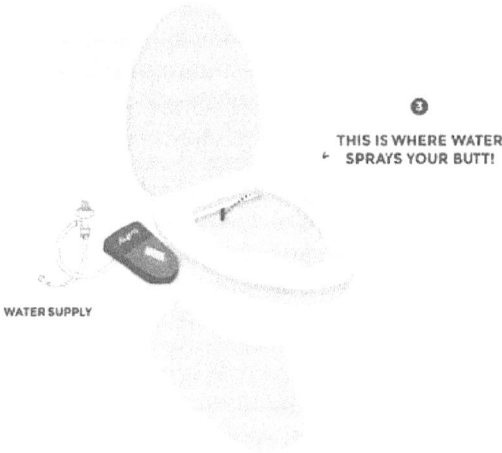

❸ THIS IS WHERE WATER
SPRAYS YOUR BUTT!

WATER SUPPLY

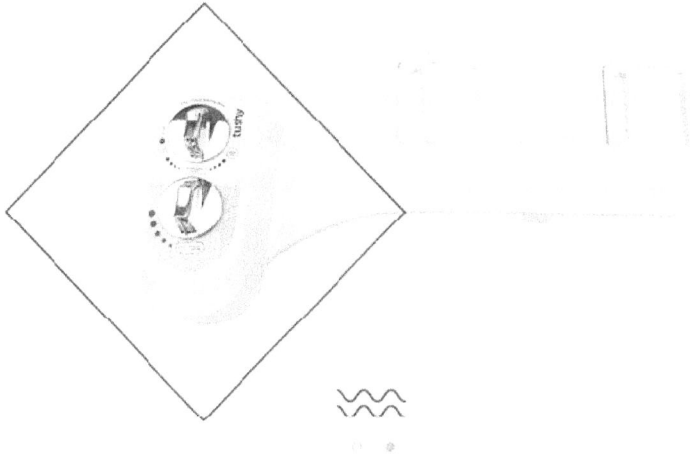

In the above picture you can see the deluxe model which comes with both a pressure control and temperature dial. Agrawal claims that the mini Bidet uses about **half a litre** of water per bowel movement. There are two types of Tushy: one that only uses cold water which retails for about $54 (£35) and one that uses warm water too for $74 (£48). Agrawal also donates a portion of all Tushy sales to organizations supporting sanitation in the developing world. So not only are you saving the planet but your also helping people. If you want to know more about this product, you can visit Tushy's website. I believe their products are also offered through the The Home Depot in Canada. There are also other manufacturer's offering a similar product including Amazetec, Brondell, Luxe, Greenco, and Toto who make the Washlet, in different price ranges, all under $80 US. Only Toto's deluxe model is about $350 US and just over $500 Canadian. Many of these are offered through Amazon so there are a lot of options for your research if you want to go high tech. Keep in mind some Plumbing knowledge will be needed or a Plumber to install as there are both cold and hot water lines to connect. The Toto Bidet has a 4.5 star rating so it must be good. Finally, if you choose to go this route, make sure your particular toilet can fit this Bidet attachment as it has to work by way of the toilet cover holes in the porcelain.

Back to top

To reach the Author to ask any questions regarding setting up your very own Towelette System or to clarify some confusion you may have, simply send an email: E-mail Trace

Also be sure to visit my Profile on Smashwords. Simply visit me at:

Trace's Smashwords Profile

Back to top

www.ingramcontent.com/pod-product-compliance
Lightning Source LLC
Chambersburg PA
CBHW030000290326
41935CB00008B/645